Diabetic Meal Prep Cookbook

Diabetic cookbook and meal plan for newly diagnosed patients delicious and comfortable recipes for a healthy lifestyle with diet plan

TABLE OF CONTENTS

BREAKFAST RECIPES

Blueberry Breakfast Cake

Preparation time: 15 minutes

Cooking time: 45 minutes

Servings: 12

Ingredients:

For the topping

- ¼ cup finely chopped walnuts

- 1/2 teaspoon ground cinnamon

- 2 tablespoons butter, chopped into small pieces

- 2 tablespoons sugar

For the cake

- Nonstick cooking spray

- 1 cup whole-wheat pastry flour

- 1 cup oat flour

- ¼ cup sugar

- 2 teaspoons baking powder

- 1 large egg, beaten

- 1/2 cup skim milk

- 2 tablespoons butter, melted

- 1 teaspoon grated lemon peel

- 2 cups fresh or frozen blueberries

Directions:

To make the topping

1. In a small bowl, stir together the walnuts, cinnamon, butter, and sugar. Set aside.

To make the cake

1. Preheat the oven to 350f. Spray a 9-inch square pan with cooking spray. Set aside.
2. In a large bowl, stir together the pastry flour, oat flour, sugar, and baking powder.
3. Add the egg, milk, butter, and lemon peel, and stir until there are no dry spots.

4. Stir in the blueberries, and gently mix until incorporated. Press the batter into the prepared pan, using a spoon to flatten it into the dish.
5. Sprinkle the topping over the cake.
6. Bake for 40 to 45 minutes, until a toothpick inserted into the cake comes out clean, and serve.

Nutrition: calories: 177; total fat: 7g; saturated fat: 3g; protein: 4g; carbs: 26g; sugar: 9g; fiber: 3g; cholesterol: 26mg; sodium: 39mg

Whole-Grain Pancakes

Preparation time: 10 minutes

Cooking time: 15 minutes

Servings: 4 to 6

Ingredients:

- 2 cups whole-wheat pastry flour

- 4 teaspoons baking powder

- 2 teaspoons ground cinnamon

- 1/2 teaspoon salt

- 2 cups skim milk, plus more as needed

- 2 large eggs

- 1 tablespoon honey

- Nonstick cooking spray

- Maple syrup, for serving

- Fresh fruit, for serving

Directions:

1. In a large bowl, stir together the flour, baking powder, cinnamon, and salt.
2. Add the milk, eggs, and honey, and stir well to combine. If needed, add more milk, 1 tablespoon at a time, until there are no dry spots and you have a pourable batter.
3. Heat a large skillet over medium-high heat, and spray it with cooking spray.
4. Using a ¼-cup measuring cup, scoop 2 or 3 pancakes into the skillet at a time. Cook for a couple of minutes, until bubbles form on the surface of the pancakes, flip, and cook for 1 to 2 minutes more, until golden brown and cooked through. Repeat with the remaining batter.
5. Serve topped with maple syrup or fresh fruit.

Nutrition: calories: 392; total fat: 4g; saturated fat: 1g; protein: 15g; carbs: 71g; sugar: 11g; fiber: 9g; cholesterol: 95mg; sodium: 396mg

Buckwheat Grouts Breakfast Bowl

Preparation time: 5 minutes, plus overnight to soak

Cooking time: 10 to 12 minutes

Servings: 4

Ingredients:

- 3 cups skim milk

- 1 cup buckwheat grouts

- ¼ cup chia seeds

- 2 teaspoons vanilla extract

- 1/2 teaspoon ground cinnamon

- Pinch salt

- 1 cup water

- 1/2 cup unsalted pistachios

- 2 cups sliced fresh strawberries

- ¼ cup cacao nibs (optional)

Directions:

1. In a large bowl, stir together the milk, groats, chia seeds, vanilla, cinnamon, and salt. Cover and refrigerate overnight.
2. The next morning, transfer the soaked mixture to a medium pot and add the water. Bring to a boil over medium-high heat, reduce the heat to maintain a simmer, and cook for 10 to 12 minutes, until the buckwheat is tender and thickened.
3. Transfer to bowls and serve, topped with the pistachios, strawberries, and cacao nibs (if using).

Nutrition: calories: 340; total fat: 8g; saturated fat: 1g; protein: 15g; carbs: 52g; sugar: 14g; fiber: 10g; cholesterol: 4mg; sodium: 140mg

Peach Muesli Bake

Preparation time: 10 minutes

Cooking time: 40 minutes

Servings: 8

Ingredients:

- Nonstick cooking spray

- 2 cups skim milk

- 11/2 cups rolled oats

- 1/2 cup chopped walnuts

- 1 large egg

- 2 tablespoons maple syrup

- 1 teaspoon ground cinnamon

- 1 teaspoon baking powder

- 1/2 teaspoon salt

- 2 to 3 peaches, sliced

Directions:

1. Preheat the oven to 375f. Spray a 9-inch square baking dish with cooking spray. Set aside.
2. In a large bowl, stir together the milk, oats, walnuts, egg, maple syrup, cinnamon, baking powder, and salt. Spread half the mixture in the prepared baking dish.
3. Place half the peaches in a single layer across the oat mixture.
4. Spread the remaining oat mixture over the top. Add the remaining peaches in a thin layer over the oats. Bake for 35 to 40 minutes, uncovered, until thickened and browned.
5. Cut into 8 squares and serve warm.

Nutrition: calories: 138; total fat: 3g; saturated fat: 1g; protein: 6g; carbs: 22g; sugar: 10g; fiber: 3g; cholesterol: 24mg; sodium: 191mg

APPETIZER RECIPES

Tomato and Roasted Cod

Preparation Time: 10 minutes

Cooking Time: 35 minutes

Serving: 2

Ingredients

- 2 (4-oz) cod fillets

- 1 cup cherry tomatoes

- 2/3 cup onion

- 2 tsp orange rind

- 1 tbsp extra virgin olive oil

- 1 tsp thyme (dried)

- 1/4 tsp salt, divided

- 1/4 tsp pepper, divided

Directions

1. Preheat oven to 400°F. Mix in half tomatoes, sliced onion, grated orange rind, extra virgin olive oil, dried thyme, and 1/8 salt and pepper. Fry 25 minutes. Remove from oven.

2. Arrange fish on pan, and flavor with remaining 1/8 tsp each salt and pepper. Put reserved tomato mixture over fish. Bake 10 minutes.

Nutrition 120 Calories 9g Protein 2g Fat

French Broccoli Salad

Preparation Time: 10 minutes,

Cooking Time: 10 minutes;

Servings: 10

Ingredients:

- 8 cups broccoli florets

- 3 strips of bacon, cooked and crumbled

- ¼ cup sunflower kernels

- 1 bunch of green onion, sliced

- What you will need from the store cupboard:

- 3 tablespoons seasoned rice vinegar

- 3 tablespoons canola oil

- 1/2 cup dried cranberries

Directions:

1. Combine the green onion, cranberries, and broccoli in a bowl.

2. Whisk the vinegar, and oil in another bowl. Blend well.

3. Now drizzle over the broccoli mix.

4. Coat well by tossing.

5. Sprinkle bacon and sunflower kernels before serving.

Nutrition: Calories 121, Carbohydrates 14g, Cholesterol 2mg, Fiber 3g, Sugar 1g, Fat 7g, Protein 3g, Sodium 233mg

Tenderloin Grilled Salad

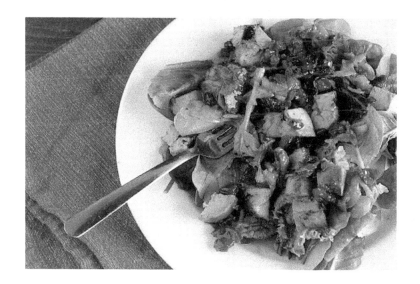

Preparation Time: 10 minutes, Cooking Time: 20 minutes; Servings: 5

Ingredients:

- 1 lb. pork tenderloin

- 10 cups mixed salad greens

- 2 oranges, seedless, cut into bite-sized pieces

- 1 tablespoon orange zest, grated

- What you will need from the store cupboard:

- 2 tablespoons of cider vinegar

- 2 tablespoons olive oil

- 2 teaspoons Dijon mustard

- 1/2 cup juice of an orange

- 2 teaspoons honey

- 1/2 teaspoon ground pepper

Directions:

1. Bring together all the dressing ingredients in a bowl.

2. Grill each side of the pork covered over medium heat for 9 minutes.

3. Slice after 5 minutes.

4. Slice the tenderloin thinly.

5. Keep the greens on your serving plate.

6. Top with the pork and oranges.

7. Sprinkle nuts (optional).

Nutrition: Calories 211, Carbohydrates 13g, Cholesterol 51mg, Fiber 3g, Sugar 0.8g, Fat 9g, Protein 20g, Sodium 113mg

Barley Veggie Salad

Preparation Time: 10 minutes,

Cooking Time: 20 minutes;

Servings: 6

Ingredients:

- 1 tomato, seeded and chopped

- 2 tablespoons parsley, minced

- 1 yellow pepper, chopped

- 1 tablespoon basil, minced

- ¼ cup almonds, toasted

- What you will need from the store cupboard:

- 1-1/4 cups vegetable broth

- 1 cup barley

- 1 tablespoon lemon juice

- 2 tablespoons of white wine vinegar

- 3 tablespoons olive oil

- ¼ teaspoon pepper

- 1/2 teaspoon salt

- 1 cup of water

Directions:

1. Boil the broth, barley, and water in a saucepan.

2. Reduce heat. Cover and let it simmer for 10 minutes.

3. Take out from the heat.

4. In the meantime, bring together the parsley, yellow pepper, and tomato in a bowl.

5. Stir the barley in.

6. Whisk the vinegar, oil, basil, lemon juice, water, pepper and salt in a bowl.

7. Pour this over your barley mix. Toss to coat well.

8. Stir the almonds in before serving.

Nutrition: Calories 211, Carbohydrates 27g, Cholesterol 0mg, Fiber 7g, Sugar 0g, Fat 10g, Protein 6g, Sodium 334mg

Spinach Shrimp Salad

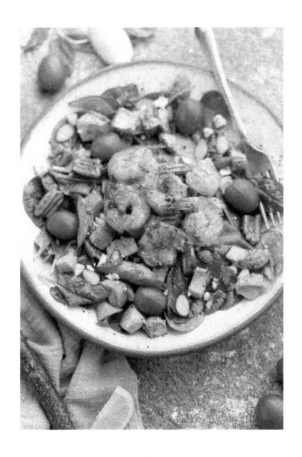

Preparation Time: 10 minutes,

Cooking Time: 10 minutes;

Servings: 4

Ingredients:

- 1 lb. uncooked shrimp, peeled and deveined

- 2 tablespoons parsley, minced

- ¾ cup halved cherry tomatoes

- 1 medium lemon

- 4 cups baby spinach

- What you will need from the store cupboard:

- 2 tablespoons butter

- 3 minced garlic cloves

- ¼ teaspoon pepper

- ¼ teaspoon salt

Directions:

1. Melt the butter over medium temperature in a nonstick skillet.

2. Add the shrimp.

3. Now cook the shrimp for 3 minutes until your shrimp becomes pink.

4. Add the parsley and garlic.

5. Cook for another minute. Take out from the heat.

6. Keep the spinach in your salad bowl.

7. Top with the shrimp mix and tomatoes.

8. Drizzle lemon juice on the salad.

9. Sprinkle pepper and salt.

Nutrition: Calories 201, Carbohydrates 6g, Cholesterol 153mg, Fiber 2g, Sugar 0g, Fat 10g, Protein 21g, Sodium 350mg

FIRST COURSE RECIPES

Chicken and Pepperoni

Preparation Time: 4 minutes

Cooking Time: 4 hours

Serving: 5

Ingredients

- 3½ to 4 pounds meaty chicken pieces

- 1/8 teaspoon salt

- 1/8 teaspoon black pepper

- 2 ounces sliced turkey pepperoni

- ¼ cup sliced pitted ripe olives

- ½ cup reduced-sodium chicken broth

- 1 tablespoon tomato paste

- 1 teaspoon dried Italian seasoning, crushed

- ½ cup shredded part-skim mozzarella cheese (2 ounces)

Direction

1. Put chicken into a 3 1/2 to 5-qt. slow cooker. Sprinkle pepper and salt on the chicken. Slice pepperoni slices in half. Put olives and pepperoni into the slow cooker. In a small bowl, blend Italian seasoning, tomato paste and chicken broth together. Transfer the mixture into the slow cooker.

2. Cook with a cover for 3-3 1/2 hours on high.

3. Transfer the olives, pepperoni and chicken onto a serving platter with a slotted spoon. Discard the cooking liquid. Sprinkle cheese over the chicken. Use foil to loosely cover and allow to sit for 5 minutes to melt the cheese.

Nutrition 243 Calories 1g Carbohydrate 41g Protein

Chicken and Sausage Gumbo

Preparation Time: 6 minutes

Cooking Time: 4 hours

Serving: 5

Ingredients

- 1/3 cup all-purpose flour

- 1 (14 ounce) can reduced-sodium chicken broth

- 2 cups chicken breast

- 8 ounces smoked turkey sausage links

- 2 cups sliced fresh okra

- 1 cup water

- 1 cup coarsely chopped onion

- 1 cup sweet pepper

- ½ cup sliced celery

- 4 cloves garlic, minced

- 1 teaspoon dried thyme

- ½ teaspoon ground black pepper

- ¼ teaspoon cayenne pepper

- 3 cups hot cooked brown rice

Direction

1. To make the roux: Cook the flour upon a medium heat in a heavy medium-sized saucepan, stirring periodically, for roughly 6 minutes or until the flour browns. Take off the heat and slightly cool, then slowly stir in the broth. Cook the roux until it bubbles and thickens up.

2. Pour the roux in a 3 1/2- or 4-quart slow cooker, then add in cayenne pepper, black pepper, thyme, garlic, celery, sweet pepper, onion, water, okra, sausage, and chicken.

3. Cook the soup covered on a high setting for 3 - 3 1/2 hours. Take the fat off the top and serve atop hot cooked brown rice.

Nutrition 230 Calories 3g Sugar 19g Protein

Chicken, Barley, and Leek Stew

Preparation Time: 10 minutes

Cooking Time: 3 hours

Serving: 2

Ingredients

- 1-pound chicken thighs

- 1 tablespoon olive oil

- 1 (49 ounce) can reduced-sodium chicken broth

- 1 cup regular barley (not quick-cooking)

- 2 medium leeks, halved lengthwise and sliced

- 2 medium carrots, thinly sliced

- 1½ teaspoons dried basil or Italian seasoning, crushed

- ¼ teaspoon cracked black pepper

Direction

1. In the big skillet, cook the chicken in hot oil till becoming brown on all sides. In the 4-5-qt. slow cooker, whisk the

pepper, dried basil, carrots, leeks, barley, chicken broth and chicken.

2. Keep covered and cooked over high heat setting for 2 – 2.5 hours or till the barley softens. As you wish, drizzle with the parsley or fresh basil prior to serving.

Nutrition 248 Calories 6g Fiber 27g Carbohydrate

SECOND COURSE RECIPES

Cauliflower Rice with Chicken

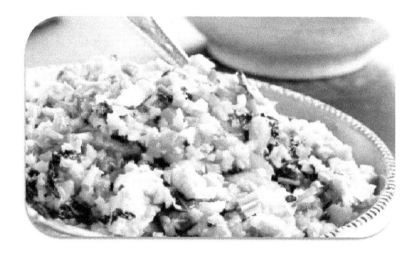

Preparation Time: 15 Minutes

Cooking Time: 15 Minutes

Servings: 4

Ingredients

- 1/2 large cauliflower

- 3/4 cup cooked meat

- 1/2 bell pepper

- 1 carrot

- 2 ribs celery

- 1 tbsp. stir fry sauce (low carb)

- 1 tbsp. extra virgin olive oil

- Salt and pepper to taste

Directions

1. Chop cauliflower in a processor to "rice." Place in a bowl.
2. Properly chop all vegetables in a food processor into thin slices.
3. Add cauliflower and other plants to WOK with heated oil. Fry until all veggies are tender.

4. Add chopped meat and sauce to the wok and fry 10 Minutes.
5. Serve.
6. This dish is very mouth-watering!

Nutrition: Calories 200 / Protein 10 g / Fat 12 g /Carbs 10 g

Turkey with Fried Eggs

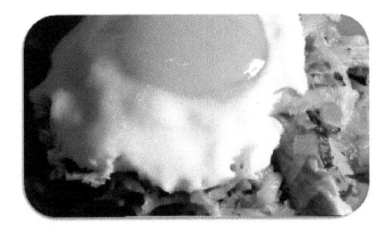

Preparation Time: 10 Minutes

Cooking Time: 20 Minutes

Servings: 4

Ingredients

- 4 large potatoes

- 1 cooked turkey thigh

- 1 large onion (about 2 cups diced)

- butter

- Chile flakes

- 4 eggs

- salt to taste

- pepper to taste

Directions

1. Rub the cold boiled potatoes on the coarsest holes of a box grater. Dice the turkey.
2. Cook the onion in as much unsalted butter as you feel comfortable with until it's just fragrant and translucent.
3. Add the rubbed potatoes and a cup of diced cooked turkey, salt and pepper to taste, and cook 20 Minutes.

Nutrition: Calories 170 / Protein 19 g / Fat 7 g / Carbs 6 g

Spiced Okra

Preparation time: 14 minutes

Cooking time: 16 minutes

Servings: 3

Ingredients:

- 2 cups okra

- ¼ teaspoon stevia

- 1 teaspoon chilli powder

- ½ teaspoon ground turmeric

- 1 tablespoon ground coriander

- 2 tablespoons fresh coriander, chopped

- 1 tablespoon ground cumin

- ¼ teaspoon salt

- 1 tablespoon desiccated coconut

- 3 tablespoons vegetable oil

- ½ teaspoon black mustard seeds

- ½ teaspoon cumin seeds

- Fresh tomatoes, to garnish

Directions:

1. Trim okra. Wash and dry.

2. Combine stevia, chilli powder, turmeric, ground coriander, fresh coriander, cumin, salt, and desiccated coconut in a bowl.

3. Heat the oil in a pan. Cook mustard and cumin seeds for 3 minutes. Stir continuously. Add okra. Tip in the spice mixture. Cook on low heat for 8 minutes.

4. Transfer to a serving dish. Garnish with fresh tomatoes.

Nutrition: Calories 163 Total Fat 4.2 g Saturated Fat 0.8 g Cholesterol 0 mg Sodium 861 mg Total Carbs 22.5 g Fiber 6.3 g Sugar 2.3 g Protein 9.2 g

Lemony Salmon Burgers

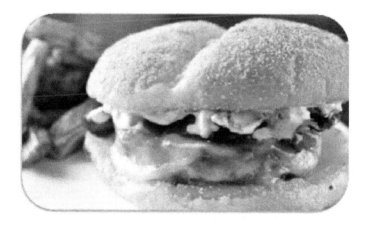

Preparation Time: 10 Minutes

Cooking Time: 10 Minutes

Servings: 4

Ingredients

- 2 (3-oz) cans boneless, skinless pink salmon

- 1/4 cup panko breadcrumbs

- 4 tsp. lemon juice

- 1/4 cup red bell pepper

- 1/4 cup sugar-free yogurt

- 1 egg

- 2 (1.5-oz) whole wheat hamburger toasted buns

Directions

1. Mix drained and flaked salmon, finely-chopped bell pepper, panko breadcrumbs.

2. Combine 2 tbsp. cup sugar-free yogurt, 3 tsp. fresh lemon juice, and egg in a bowl. Shape mixture into 2 (3-inch) patties, bake on the skillet over medium heat 4 to 5 Minutes per side.

3. Stir together 2 tbsp. sugar-free yogurt and 1 tsp. lemon juice; spread over bottom halves of buns.

4. Top each with 1 patty, and cover with bun tops.

Nutrition: Calories 131 / Protein 12 / Fat 1 g / Carbs 19 g

Caprese Turkey Burgers

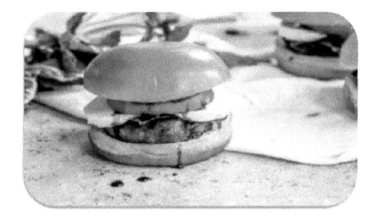

Preparation Time 10 Minutes

Cooking Time: 10 Minutes

Servings: 4

Ingredients

- 1/2 lb. 93% lean ground turkey

- 2 (1,5-oz) whole wheat hamburger buns (toasted)

- 1/4 cup shredded mozzarella cheese (part-skim)

- 1 egg

- 1 big tomato

- 1 small clove garlic

- 4 large basil leaves

- 1/8 tsp. salt

- 1/8 tsp. pepper

Directions

1. Combine turkey, white egg, Minced garlic, salt, and pepper (mix until combined);

2. Shape into 2 cutlets. Put cutlets into a skillet; cook 5 to 7 Minutes per side.

3. Top cutlets properly with cheese and sliced tomato at the end of cooking.

4. Put 1 cutlet on the bottom of each bun.

5. Top each patty with 2 basil leaves. Cover with bun tops.

Nutrition: Calories 180 / Protein 7 g / Fat 4 g / Carbs 20 g

SIDE DISH RECIPES

Low Fat Roasties

Preparation Time: 8 minutes

Cooking Time: 25 minutes

Servings: 2

Ingredients:

- 1lb roasting potatoes

- 1 garlic clove

- 1 cup vegetable stock

- 2tbsp olive oil

Directions:

1. 1.Position potatoes in the steamer basket and add the stock into the Instant Pot.
2. 2.Steam the potatoes in your Instant Pot for 15 minutes.
3. 3.Depressurize and pour away the remaining stock.
4. 4.Set to sauté and add the oil, garlic, and potatoes. Cook until brown.

Nutrition: 201 Calories 3g Carbohydrates 6g Fat

Roasted Parsnips

Preparation Time: 9 minutes

Cooking Time: 25 minutes

Servings: 2

Ingredients:

- 1lb parsnips

- 1 cup vegetable stock

- 2tbsp herbs

- 2tbsp olive oil

Directions:

1. 1.Put the parsnips in the steamer basket and add the stock into the Instant Pot.
2. 2.Steam the parsnips in your Instant Pot for 15 minutes.
3. 3.Depressurize and pour away the remaining stock.
4. 4.Set to sauté and add the oil, herbs and parsnips.
5. 5.Cook until golden and crisp.

Nutrition: 130 Calories 14g Carbohydrates 4g Protein

Lower Carb Hummus

Preparation Time: 9 minutes

Cooking Time: 60 minutes

Servings: 2

Ingredients:

- 0.5 cup dry chickpeas

- 1 cup vegetable stock

- 1 cup pumpkin puree

- 2tbsp smoked paprika

- salt and pepper to taste

Directions:

1. 1.Soak the chickpeas overnight.
2. 2.Place the chickpeas and stock in the Instant Pot.
3. 3.Cook on Beans 60 minutes.
4. 4.Depressurize naturally.
5. 5.Blend the chickpeas with the remaining ingredients.

Nutrition: 135 Calories 18g Carbohydrates 3g Fat

Sweet and Sour Red Cabbage

Preparation Time: 7 minutes

Cooking Time: 10 minutes

Servings: 8

Ingredients:

- 2 cups Spiced Pear Applesauce

- 1 small onion, chopped

- ½ cup apple cider vinegar

- ½ teaspoon kosher salt

- 1 head red cabbage

Directions:

1. 1.In the electric pressure cooker, combine the applesauce, onion, vinegar, salt, and cup of water. Stir in the cabbage.
2. 2.Seal lid of the pressure cooker.
3. 3.Cook on high pressure for 10 minutes.
4. 4.When the cooking is complete, hit Cancel and quick release the pressure.
5. 5.Once the pin drops, unlock and remove the lid.
6. 6.Spoon into a bowl or platter and serve.

Nutrition: 91 Calories 18g Carbohydrates 4g Fiber

SOUP & STEW

Dill Celery Soup

Preparation time: 10 minutes

Cooking time: 30 minutes

Servings: 4

Ingredients:

- 6 cups celery stalk, chopped

- 2 cups filtered alkaline water

- 1 medium onion, chopped

- 1/2 tsp. dill

- 1 cup of coconut milk

- 1/4 tsp. sea salt

Directions:

1. Combine all elements into the direct pot and mix fine.

2. Cover pot with lid and select soup mode it takes 30 minutes.

3. Release pressure using the quick release **Directions**: than open lid carefully.

4. Blend the soup utilizing a submersion blender until smooth.

5. Stir well and serve.

Nutrition: Calories 193 Fat 15.3 g Carbohydrates 10.9 g Protein 5.2 g Sugar 5.6 g Cholesterol 0 mg

Creamy Avocado-Broccoli Soup

Preparation time: 10 minutes

Cooking time: 15 minutes

Servings: 1-2

Ingredients:

- 2-3 flowers broccoli

- 1 small avocado

- 1 yellow onion

- 1 green or red pepper

- 1 celery stalk

- 2 cups vegetable broth (yeast-free)

- Celtic Sea Salt to taste

Directions:

1. Warmth vegetable stock (don't bubble). Include hacked onion and broccoli, and warm for a few minutes. At that point put in blender, include the avocado, pepper and celery and Blend until the soup is smooth (include some

more water whenever wanted). Flavor and serve warm. Delicious!!

Nutrition: Calories: 60g Carbohydrates: 11g Fat: 2 g Protein: 2g

Fresh Garden Vegetable Soup

Preparation time: 7 minutes

Cooking time: 20 minutes

Servings: 1-2

Ingredients:

- 2 huge carrots

- 1 little zucchini

- 1 celery stem

- 1 cup of broccoli

- 3 stalks of asparagus

- 1 yellow onion

- 1 quart of (antacid) water

- 4-5 tsps. Of sans yeast vegetable stock

- 1 tsp. new basil

- 2 tsps. Ocean salt to taste

Directions:

1. Put water in pot, include the vegetable stock just as the onion and bring to bubble.

2. In the meantime, cleave the zucchini, the broccoli and the asparagus, and shred the carrots and the celery stem in a food processor.

3. When the water is bubbling, it would be ideal if you turn off the oven as we would prefer not to heat up the vegetables. Simply put them all in the high temp water and hold up until the vegetables arrive at wanted delicacy.

4. Permit to cool somewhat, at that point put all fixings into blender and blend until you get a thick, smooth consistency.

Nutrition: Calories: 43 Carbohydrates: 7g Fat: 1 g

Raw Some Gazpacho Soup

Preparation time: 7 minutes

Cooking time: 3 hours

Servings: 3-4

Ingredients:

- 500g tomatoes

- 1 small cucumber

- 1 red pepper

- 1 onion

- 2 cloves of garlic

- 1 small chili

- 1 quart of water (preferably alkaline water)

- 4 tbsp. cold-pressed olive oil

- Juice of one fresh lemon

- 1 dash of cayenne pepper

- Sea salt to taste

Directions:

1. Remove the skin of the cucumber and cut all vegetables in large pieces.

2. Put all **Ingredients** except the olive oil in a blender and mix until smooth.

3. Add the olive oil and mix again until oil is emulsified.

4. Put the soup in the fridge and chill for at least 2 hours (soup should be served ice cold).

5. Add some salt and pepper to taste, mix, place the soup in bowls, garnish with chopped scallions, cucumbers, tomatoes and peppers and enjoy!

Nutrition: Calories: 39 Carbohydrates: 8g Fat: 0.5 g Protein: 0.2g

Alkaline Carrot Soup with Fresh Mushrooms

Preparation time: 10 minutes

Cooking time: 20 minutes

Servings: 1-2

Ingredients:

- 4 mid-sized carrots

- 4 mid-sized potatoes

- 10 enormous new mushrooms (champignons or chanterelles)

- 1/2 white onion

- 2 tbsp. olive oil (cold squeezed, additional virgin)

- 3 cups vegetable stock

- 2 tbsp. parsley, new and cleaved

- Salt and new white pepper

Directions:

1. Wash and strip carrots and potatoes and dice them.

2. Warm up vegetable stock in a pot on medium heat. Cook carrots and potatoes for around 15 minutes. Meanwhile finely shape onion and braise them in a container with olive oil for around 3 minutes.

3. Wash mushrooms, slice them to wanted size and add to the container, cooking approx. an additional 5 minutes, blending at times. Blend carrots, vegetable stock and potatoes, and put substance of the skillet into pot.

4. When nearly done, season with parsley, salt and pepper and serve hot. Appreciate this alkalizing soup!

Nutrition: Calories: 75 Carbohydrates: 13g Fat: 1.8g Protein: 1 g

DESSERT

Peanut Butter Cups

Preparation Time: 5 minutes

Cooking Time: 10 minutes

Servings: 4

Ingredients:

- 1 packet plain gelatin

- ¼ cup sugar substitute

- 2 cups nonfat cream

- ½ teaspoon vanilla

- ¼ cup low-fat peanut butter

- 2 tablespoons unsalted peanuts, chopped

Directions:

1. 1.Mix gelatin, sugar substitute and cream in a pan.
2. 2.Let sit for 5 minutes.

3. 3.Place over medium heat and cook until gelatin has been dissolved.
4. 4.Stir in vanilla and peanut butter.
5. 5.Pour into custard cups. Chill for 3 hours.
6. 6.Top with the peanuts and serve.

Nutrition: 171 Calories 21g Carbohydrate 6.8g Protein

Fruit Pizza

Preparation Time: 5 minutes

Cooking Time: 10 minutes

Servings: 4

Ingredients:

- 1 teaspoon maple syrup

- ¼ teaspoon vanilla extract

- ½ cup coconut milk yogurt

- 2 round slices watermelon

- ½ cup blackberries, sliced

- ½ cup strawberries, sliced

- 2 tablespoons coconut flakes (unsweetened)

Directions:

1. 1.Mix maple syrup, vanilla and yogurt in a bowl.
2. 2.Spread the mixture on top of the watermelon slice.
3. 3.Top with the berries and coconut flakes.

Nutrition: 70 Calories 14.6g Carbohydrate 1.2g Protein

Choco Peppermint Cake

Preparation Time: 5 minutes

Cooking Time: 10 minutes

Servings: 4

Ingredients:

- Cooking spray
- 1/3 cup oil
- 15 oz. package chocolate cake mix
- 3 eggs, beaten
- 1 cup water
- ¼ teaspoon peppermint extract

Directions:

1. 1.Spray slow cooker with oil.
2. 2.Mix all the ingredients in a bowl.
3. 3.Use an electric mixer on medium speed setting to mix ingredients for 2 minutes.
4. 4.Pour mixture into the slow cooker.
5. 5.Cover the pot and cook on low for 3 hours.
6. 6.Let cool before slicing and serving.

Nutrition: 185 Calories 27g Carbohydrate 3.8g Protein

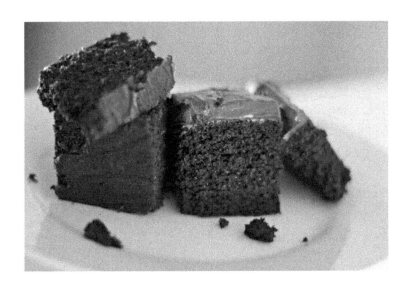

Roasted Mango

Preparation Time: 5 minutes

Cooking Time: 10 minutes

Servings: 4

Ingredients:

- 2 mangoes, sliced

- 2 teaspoons crystallized ginger, chopped

- 2 teaspoons orange zest

- 2 tablespoons coconut flakes (unsweetened)

Directions:

1. 1.Preheat your oven to 350 degrees F.
2. 2.Add mango slices in custard cups.
3. 3.Top with the ginger, orange zest and coconut flakes.
4. 4.Bake in the oven for 10 minutes.

Nutrition: 89 Calories 20g Carbohydrate 0.8g Protein

Roasted Plums

Preparation Time: 5 minutes

Cooking Time: 10 minutes

Servings: 4

Ingredients:

- Cooking spray
- 6 plums, sliced
- ½ cup pineapple juice (unsweetened)
- 1 tablespoon brown sugar
- 2 tablespoons brown sugar
- ¼ teaspoon ground cardamom
- ½ teaspoon ground cinnamon
- 1/8 teaspoon ground cumin

Directions:

1. 1.Combine all the ingredients in a baking pan.
2. 2.Roast in the oven at 450 degrees F for 20 minutes.

Nutrition: 102 Calories 18.7g Carbohydrate 2g Protein

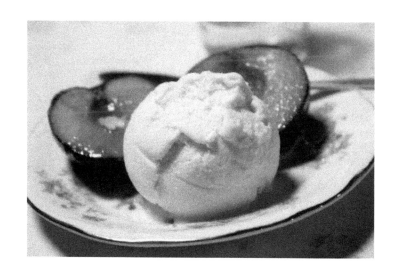

Figs with Honey & Yogurt

Preparation Time: 5 minutes

Cooking Time: 10 minutes

Servings: 4

Ingredients:

- ½ teaspoon vanilla

- 8 oz. nonfat yogurt

- 2 figs, sliced

- 1 tablespoon walnuts, chopped and toasted

- 2 teaspoons honey

Directions:

1. 1.Stir vanilla into yogurt.
2. 2.Mix well.
3. 3.Top with the figs and sprinkle with walnuts.
4. 4.Drizzle with honey and serve.

Nutrition: 157 Calories 24g Carbohydrate 7g Protein

Flourless Chocolate Cake

Preparation Time: 10 minutes

Cooking Time: 45 minutes

Servings: 6

Ingredients:

- ½ Cup of stevia

- 12 Ounces of unsweetened baking chocolate

- 2/3 Cup of ghee

- 1/3 Cup of warm water

- ¼ Teaspoon of salt

- 4 Large pastured eggs

- 2 Cups of boiling water

Directions:

1. 1.Line the bottom of a 9-inch pan of a spring form with a parchment paper.
2. 2.Heat the water in a small pot; then add the salt and the stevia over the water until wait until the mixture becomes completely dissolved.

3. 3.Melt the baking chocolate into a double boiler or simply microwave it for about 30 seconds.
4. 4.Mix the melted chocolate and the butter in a large bowl with an electric mixer.
5. 5.Beat in your hot mixture; then crack in the egg and whisk after adding each of the eggs.
6. 6.Pour the obtained mixture into your prepared spring form tray.
7. 7.Wrap the spring form tray with a foil paper.
8. 8.Place the spring form tray in a large cake tray and add boiling water right to the outside; make sure the depth doesn't exceed 1 inch.
9. 9.Bake the cake into the water bath for about 45 minutes at a temperature of about 350 F.
10. 10.Remove the tray from the boiling water and transfer to a wire to cool.
11. 11.Let the cake chill for an overnight in the refrigerator.

Nutrition 295 Calories 6g Carbohydrates 4g Fiber

Lava Cake

Preparation Time: 10 minutes

Cooking Time: 10 minutes

Servings: 2

Ingredients:

- 2 Oz of dark chocolate; you should at least use chocolate of 85% cocoa solids

- 1 Tablespoon of super-fine almond flour

- 2 Oz of unsalted almond butter

- 2 Large eggs

Directions:

1. 1.Heat your oven to a temperature of about 350 Fahrenheit.
2. 2.Grease 2 heat proof ramekins with almond butter.
3. 3.Now, melt the chocolate and the almond butter and stir very well.
4. 4.Beat the eggs very well with a mixer.
5. 5.Add the eggs to the chocolate and the butter mixture and mix very well with almond flour and the swerve; then stir.

6. 6.Pour the dough into 2 ramekins.
7. 7.Bake for about 9 to 10 minutes.
8. 8.Turn the cakes over plates and serve with pomegranate seeds!

Nutrition 459 Calories 3.5g Carbohydrates 0.8g Fiber

JUICE AND SMOOTHIE RECIPES

Dandelion Avocado Smoothie

Preparation time: 15 minutes

Cooking time: 0

Servings: 1

Ingredients:

- One cup of Dandelion

- One Orange (juiced)

- Coconut water

- One Avocado

- One key lime (juice)

Directions:

1. In a high-speed blender until smooth, blend **Ingredients**.

Nutrition: Calories: 160 Fat: 15 grams Carbohydrates: 9 grams
Protein: 2 grams

Amaranth Greens and Avocado Smoothie

Preparation time: 15 minutes

Cooking time: 0

Servings: 1

Ingredients:

- One key lime (juice).

- Two sliced apples (seeded).

- Half avocado.

- Two cupsful of amaranth greens.

- Two cupsful of watercress.

- One cupful of water.

Directions:

1. Add the whole recipes together and transfer them into the blender. Blend thoroughly until smooth.

Nutrition: Calories: 160 Fat: 15 grams Carbohydrates: 9 grams Protein: 2 grams

Lettuce, Orange and Banana Smoothie

Preparation time: 15 minutes

Cooking time: 0

Servings: 1

Ingredients:

- One and a half cupsful of fresh lettuce.

- One large banana.

- One cup of mixed berries of your choice.

- One juiced orange.

Directions:

1. First, add the orange juice to your blender.

2. Add the remaining recipes and blend thoroughly.

3. Enjoy the rest of your day.

Nutrition: Calories: 252.1 Protein: 4.1 g

Delicious Elderberry Smoothie

Preparation time: 15 minutes

Cooking time: 0

Servings: 1

Ingredients:

- One cupful of Elderberry

- One cupful of Cucumber

- One large apple

- A quarter cupful of water

Directions:

1. Add the whole recipes together into a blender. Grind very well until they are uniformly smooth and enjoy.

Nutrition: Calories: 106 Carbohydrates: 26.68

Peaches Zucchini Smoothie

Preparation time: 15 minutes

Cooking time: 0

Servings: 1

Ingredients:

- A half cupful of squash.

- A half cupful of peaches.

- A quarter cupful of coconut water.

- A half cupful of Zucchini.

Directions:

1. Add the whole recipes together into a blender and blend until smooth and serve.

Nutrition: 55 Calories 0g Fat 2g Of Protein 10mg Sodium14 G Carbohydrate 2g Of Fiber

Ginger Orange and Strawberry Smoothie

Preparation time: 15 minutes

Cooking time: 0

Servings: 1

Ingredients:

- One cup of strawberry.

- One large orange (juice)

- One large banana.

- Quarter small sized ginger (peeled and sliced).

Directions:

2. Transfer the orange juice to a clean blender.

3. Add the remaining recipes and blend thoroughly until smooth.

4. Enjoy. Wow! You have ended the 9th day of your weight loss and detox journey.

Nutrition: 32 Calories 0.3g Fat 2g Of Protei 10mg Sodium 14g Carbohydrate Water2g Of Fiber.

Kale Parsley and Chia Seeds Detox Smoothie

Preparation time: 15 minutes

Cooking time: 0

Servings: 1

Ingredients:

- Three tbsp. chia seeds (grounded).

- One cupful of water.

- One sliced banana.

- One pear (chopped).

- One cupful of organic kale.

- One cupful of parsley.

- Two tbsp. of lemon juice.

- A dash of cinnamon.

Directions:

1. Add the whole recipes together into a blender and pour the water before blending. Blend at high speed until smooth and enjoy. You may or may not place it in the

refrigerator depending on how hot or cold the weather appears.

Nutrition: 75 calories 1g fat 5g protein 10g fiber

Watermelon Limenade

Preparation time: 5 Minutes

Cooking time: 0 minutes

Servings: 6

When it comes to refreshing summertime drinks, lemonade is always near the top of the list. This Watermelon "Limenade" is perfect for using up leftover watermelon or for those early fall days when stores and farmers are almost giving them away. You can also substitute 4 cups of ice for the cold water to create a delicious summertime slushy.

Ingredients

- 4 cups diced watermelon

- 4 cups cold water

- 2 tablespoons freshly squeezed lemon juice

- 1 tablespoon freshly squeezed lime juice

Directions

1. In a blender, combine the watermelon, water, lemon juice, and lime juice, and blend for 1 minute.

2. Strain the contents through a fine-mesh sieve or nut-milk bag. Serve chilled. Store in the refrigerator for up to 3 days.

SERVING TIP: Slice up a few lemon or lime wedges to serve with your Watermelon Limenade, or top it with a few fresh mint leaves to give it an extra-crisp, minty flavor.

Nutrition Calories: 60

Bubbly Orange Soda

Preparation time: 5 Minutes

Cooking time: 0 minutes

Servings: 4

Soda can be one of the toughest things to give up when you first adopt a WFPB diet. That's partially because refined sugars and caffeine are addictive, but it can also be because carbonated beverages are fun to drink! With sweetness from the orange juice and bubbliness from the carbonated water, this orange "soda" is perfect for assisting in the transition from SAD to WFPB.

Ingredients

- 4 cups carbonated water

- 2 cups pulp-free orange juice (4 oranges, freshly squeezed and strained)

Directions

1. For each serving, pour 2 parts carbonated water and 1-part orange juice over ice right before serving.

2. Stir and enjoy.

SERVING TIP: This recipe is best made right before drinking. The amount of fizz in the carbonated water will decrease the longer it's open, so if you're going to make it ahead of time, make sure it's stored in an airtight, refrigerator-safe container.

Nutrition Calories: 56

Creamy Cashew Milk

Preparation time: 5 Minutes

Cooking time: 0 minutes

Servings: 8

Learning how to make your own plant-based milks can be one of the best ways to save money and ditch dairy for good. This is one of the easiest milk recipes to master, and if you have a high-speed blender, you can skip the straining step and go straight to a refrigerator-safe container. Large mason jars work great for storing plant-based milk, as they allow you to give a quick shake before each use.

Ingredients

- 4 cups water

- ¼ cup raw cashews, soaked overnight

Directions

1. In a blender, blend the water and cashews on high speed for 2 minutes.

2. Strain with a nut-milk bag or cheesecloth, then store in the refrigerator for up to 5 days.

VARIATION TIP: This recipe makes unsweetened cashew milk that can be used in savory and sweet dishes. For a creamier version to put in your coffee, cut the amount of water in half. For a sweeter version, add 1 to 2 tablespoons maple syrup and 1 teaspoon vanilla extract before blending.

Nutrition Calories: 18

Homemade Oat Milk

Preparation time: 5 Minutes

Cooking time: 0 minutes

Servings: 8

Oat milk is a fantastic option if you need a nut-free milk or just want an extremely inexpensive plant-based milk. Making a half-gallon jar at home costs a fraction of the price of other plant-based or dairy milks. Oat milk can be used in both savory and sweet dishes.

Ingredients

- 1 cup rolled oats

- 4 cups water

Directions

1. Put the oats in a medium bowl, and cover with cold water. Soak for 15 minutes, then drain and rinse the oats.

2. Pour the cold water and the soaked oats into a blender. Blend for 60 to 90 seconds, or just until the mixture is a creamy white color throughout. (Blending any further may over blend the oats, resulting in a gummy milk.)

3. Strain through a nut-milk bag or colander, then store in the refrigerator for up to 5 days.

Nutrition Calories: 39

OTHER DIABETIC RECIPES

Scallion Sandwich

Preparation Time: 10 minutes

Cooking Time: 10 minutes

Servings: 1

Ingredients:

- 2 slices wheat bread

- 2 teaspoons butter, low fat

- 2 scallions, sliced thinly

- 1 tablespoon of parmesan cheese, grated

- 3/4 cup of cheddar cheese, reduced fat, grated

Directions:

1. Preheat the Air fryer to 356 degrees.

2. Spread butter on a slice of bread. Place inside the cooking basket with the butter side facing down.

3. Place cheese and scallions on top. Spread the rest of the butter on the other slice of bread Put it on top of the sandwich and sprinkle with parmesan cheese.

4. Cook for 10 minutes.

Nutrition: Calorie: 154Carbohydrate: 9g Fat: 2.5g Protein: 8.6g Fiber: 2.4g

Lean Lamb and Turkey Meatballs with Yogurt

Preparation Time: 10 minutes

Servings: 4

Cooking Time: 8 minutes

Ingredients:

- 1 egg white

- 4 ounces ground lean turkey

- 1 pound of ground lean lamb

- 1 teaspoon each of cayenne pepper, ground coriander, red chili pastes, salt, and ground cumin

- 2 garlic cloves, minced

- 1 1/2 tablespoons parsley, chopped

- 1 tablespoon mint, chopped

- 1/4 cup of olive oil

For the yogurt

- 2 tablespoons of buttermilk

- 1 garlic clove, minced

- 1/4 cup mint, chopped

- 1/2 cup of Greek yogurt, non-fat

- Salt to taste

Directions:

1. Set the Air Fryer to 390 degrees.

2. Mix all the ingredients for the meatballs in a bowl. Roll and mold them into golf-size round pieces. Arrange in the cooking basket. Cook for 8 minutes.

3. While waiting, combine all the ingredients for the mint yogurt in a bowl. Mix well.

4. Serve the meatballs with the mint yogurt. Top with olives and fresh mint.

Nutrition: Calorie: 154 Carbohydrate: 9g Fat: 2.5g Protein: 8.6g Fiber: 2.4g

Air Fried Section and Tomato

Preparation Time: 10 minutes

Cooking Time: 5 minutes

Servings: 2

Ingredients:

- 1 aubergine, sliced thickly into 4 disks

- 1 tomato, sliced into 2 thick disks

- 2 tsp. feta cheese, reduced fat

- 2 fresh basil leaves, minced

- 2 balls, small buffalo mozzarella, reduced fat, roughly torn

- Pinch of salt

- Pinch of black pepper

Directions:

1. Preheat Air Fryer to 330 degrees F.

2. Spray small amount of oil into the Air fryer basket. Fry aubergine slices for 5 minutes or until golden brown on both sides. Transfer to a plate.

3. Fry tomato slices in batches for 5 minutes or until seared on both sides.

4. To serve, stack salad starting with an aborigine base, buffalo mozzarella, basil leaves, tomato slice, and 1/2-teaspoon feta cheese.

5. Top of with another slice of aborigine and 1/2 tsp. feta cheese. Serve.

Nutrition: Calorie: 140.3Carbohydrate: 26.6Fat: 3.4g Protein: 4.2g Fiber: 7.3g

Cheesy Salmon Fillets

Preparation Time: 15 minutes

Cooking Time: 20 minutes

Servings: 2-3

Ingredients: For the salmon fillets

- 2 pieces, 4 oz. each salmon fillets, choose even cuts

- 1/2 cup sour cream, reduced fat

- ¼ cup cottage cheese, reduced fat

- ¼ cup Parmigiano-Reggiano cheese, freshly grated

Garnish:

- Spanish paprika

- 1/2-piece lemon, cut into wedges

Directions:

1. Preheat Air Fryer to 330 degrees F.

2. To make the salmon fillets, mix sour cream, cottage cheese, and Parmigiano-Reggiano cheese in a bowl.

3. Layer salmon fillets in the Air fryer basket. Fry for 20 minutes or until cheese turns golden brown.

4. To assemble, place a salmon fillet and sprinkle paprika. Garnish with lemon wedges and squeeze lemon juice on top. Serve.

Nutrition: Calorie: 274Carbohydrate: 1g Fat: 19g Protein: 24g Fiber: 0.5g

Salmon with Asparagus

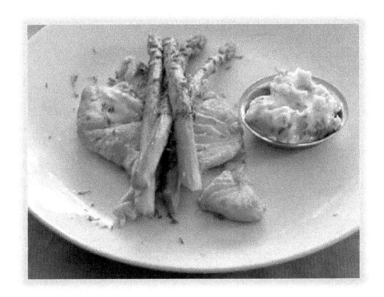

Preparation Time: 5 Minutes

Cooking Time: 10 Minutes

Servings: 3

Ingredients:

- 1 lb. Salmon, sliced into fillets

- 1 tbsp. Olive Oil

- Salt & Pepper, as needed

- 1 bunch of Asparagus, trimmed

- 2 cloves of Garlic, minced

- Zest & Juice of 1/2 Lemon

- 1 tbsp. Butter, salted

Directions:

1. Spoon in the butter and olive oil into a large pan and heat it over medium-high heat.

2. Once it becomes hot, place the salmon and season it with salt and pepper.

3. Cook for 4 minutes per side and then cook the other side.

4. Stir in the garlic and lemon zest to it.

5. Cook for further 2 minutes or until slightly browned.

6. Off the heat and squeeze the lemon juice over it.

7. Serve it hot.

Nutrition: Calories: 409Kcal Carbohydrates: 2.7g Proteins: 32.8g Fat: 28.8g Sodium: 497mg

Shrimp in Garlic Butter

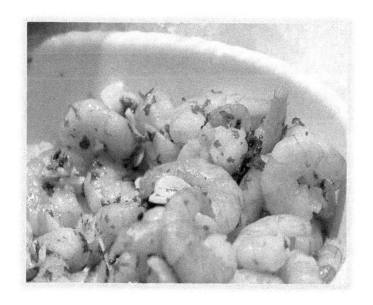

Preparation Time: 5 Minutes

Cooking Time: 20 Minutes

Servings: 4

Ingredients:

- 1 lb. Shrimp, peeled & deveined

- ¼ tsp. Red Pepper Flakes

- 6 tbsp. Butter, divided

- 1/2 cup Chicken Stock

- Salt & Pepper, as needed

- 2 tbsp. Parsley, minced

- 5 cloves of Garlic, minced

- 2 tbsp. Lemon Juice

Directions:

1. Heat a large bottomed skillet over medium-high heat.

2. Spoon in two tablespoons of the butter and melt it. Add the shrimp.

3. Season it with salt and pepper. Sear for 4 minutes or until shrimp gets cooked.

4. Transfer the shrimp to a plate and stir in the garlic.

5. Sauté for 30 seconds or until aromatic.

6. Pour the chicken stock and whisk it well. Allow it to simmer for 5 to 10 minutes or until it has reduced to half.

7. Spoon the remaining butter, red pepper, and lemon juice to the sauce. Mix.

8. Continue cooking for another 2 minutes.

9. Take off the pan from the heat and add the cooked shrimp to it.

10. Garnish with parsley and transfer to the serving bowl.

11. Enjoy.

Nutrition: Calories: 307Kcal Carbohydrates: 3g Proteins: 27g Fat: 20g Sodium: 522mg

Cobb Salad

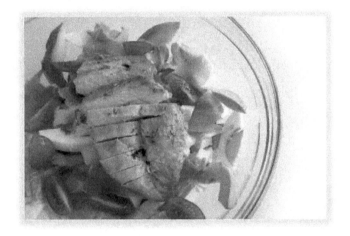

Keto & Under 30 Minutes

Preparation Time: 5 Minutes

Cooking Time: 5 Minutes

Servings: 1

Ingredients:

- 4 Cherry Tomatoes, chopped

- ¼ cup Bacon, cooked & crumbled

- 1/2 of 1 Avocado, chopped

- 2 oz. Chicken Breast, shredded

- 1 Egg, hardboiled

- 2 cups Mixed Green salad

- 1 oz. Feta Cheese, crumbled

Directions:

1. Toss all the ingredients for the Cobb salad in a large mixing bowl and toss well.

2. Serve and enjoy it.

Nutrition: Calories: 307Kcal Carbohydrates: 3g Proteins: 27g Fat: 20g Sodium: 522mg

CPSIA information can be obtained
at www.ICGtesting.com
Printed in the USA
BVHW080323040521
606354BV00010B/975